I0842416

Breakfast

Recipe:

Serving: Prep Time:

Cook Time: Temperature:

Ingredients: Methods:

Wine Pairing:

From the Kitchen of:

Recipe:

Serving: Prep Time:

Cook Time: Temperature:

Ingredients: Methods:

Wine Pairing:

From the Kitchen of:

Recipe:

Serving: Prep Time:

Cook Time: Temperature:

Ingredients: Methods:

Wine Pairing:

From the Kitchen of:

Recipe:

Serving: Prep Time:

Cook Time: Temperature:

Ingredients: Methods:

Recipe:

Serving:

Prep Time:

Cook Time:

Temperature:

Ingredients:

Methods:

Wine Pairing:

From the Kitchen of:

Recipe:

Serving:

Prep Time:

Cook Time:

Temperature:

Ingredients:

Methods:

Wine Pairing:

From the Kitchen of:

Recipe:

Serving: Prep Time:

Cook Time: Temperature:

Ingredients: Methods:

Wine Pairing:

From the Kitchen of:

Recipe:

Serving:

Prep Time:

Cook Time:

Temperature:

Ingredients:

Methods:

Wine Pairing:

From the Kitchen of:

Recipe:

Serving: Prep Time:

Cook Time: Temperature:

Ingredients: Methods:

Wine Pairing:

From the Kitchen of:

Lunch

Recipe:

Serving:

Prep Time:

Cook Time:

Temperature:

Ingredients:

Methods:

Wine Pairing:

From the Kitchen of:

Recipe:

Serving: Prep Time:

Cook Time: Temperature:

Ingredients: Methods:

Wine Pairing:

From the Kitchen of:

Recipe:

Serving: Prep Time:

Cook Time: Temperature:

Ingredients: Methods:

Wine Pairing:

From the Kitchen of:

Recipe:

Serving: Prep Time:

Cook Time: Temperature:

Ingredients: Methods:

Wine Pairing:

From the Kitchen of:

Recipe: _______________________

Serving: _______________ Prep Time: _______________

Cook Time: _______________ Temperature: _______________

Ingredients:

____

____

____

____

____

____

____

____

____

____

____

____

____

____

Methods:

____

____

____

____

____

____

____

____

____

____

____

____

____

____

Wine Pairing: _______________________

From the Kitchen of: _______________________

Recipe:

Serving:

Prep Time:

Cook Time:

Temperature:

Ingredients:

Methods:

Wine Pairing:

From the Kitchen of:

Recipe:

Serving: Prep Time:

Cook Time: Temperature:

Ingredients: Methods:

Wine Pairing:

From the Kitchen of:

Recipe:

Serving: Prep Time:

Cook Time: Temperature:

Ingredients: Methods:

Wine Pairing:

From the Kitchen of:

Recipe:

Serving: Prep Time:

Cook Time: Temperature:

Ingredients: Methods:

Wine Pairing:

From the Kitchen of:

Dinner

Recipe:

Serving:

Prep Time:

Cook Time:

Temperature:

Ingredients:

Methods:

Wine Pairing:

From the Kitchen of:

Recipe:

Serving: Prep Time:

Cook Time: Temperature:

Ingredients: Methods:

Wine Pairing:

From the Kitchen of:

Recipe: _______________________________

Serving: _______________ Prep Time: _______________

Cook Time: _______________ Temperature: _______________

Ingredients:

____

____

____

____

____

____

____

____

____

____

____

____

____

____

Methods:

____

____

____

____

____

____

____

____

____

____

____

____

____

____

Wine Pairing: _______________________________

From the Kitchen of: _______________________________

Recipe:

Serving:

Prep Time:

Cook Time:

Temperature:

Ingredients:

Methods:

Wine Pairing:

From the Kitchen of:

Recipe:

Serving: Prep Time:

Cook Time: Temperature:

Ingredients: Methods:

Wine Pairing:

From the Kitchen of:

Recipe:

Serving:

Prep Time:

Cook Time:

Temperature:

Ingredients:

Methods:

Wine Pairing:

From the Kitchen of:

Recipe:

Serving:

Prep Time:

Cook Time:

Temperature:

Ingredients:

Methods:

Wine Pairing:

From the Kitchen of:

Recipe:

Serving: Prep Time:

Cook Time: Temperature:

Ingredients: Methods:

Wine Pairing:

From the Kitchen of:

Recipe:

Serving:

Prep Time:

Cook Time:

Temperature:

Ingredients:

Methods:

Wine Pairing:

From the Kitchen of:

Desserts

Recipe:

Serving:

Prep Time:

Cook Time:

Temperature:

Ingredients:

Methods:

Wine Pairing:

From the Kitchen of:

Recipe: _______________________

Serving: _______________ Prep Time: _______________

Cook Time: _______________ Temperature: _______________

Ingredients:

____

____

____

____

____

____

____

____

____

____

____

____

____

____

____

Methods:

____

____

____

____

____

____

____

____

____

____

____

____

____

____

Wine Pairing: _______________________________________

From the Kitchen of: _______________________________________

Recipe:

Serving: Prep Time:

Cook Time: Temperature:

Ingredients: Methods:

Wine Pairing:

From the Kitchen of:

Recipe:

Serving:

Prep Time:

Cook Time:

Temperature:

Ingredients:

Methods:

Wine Pairing:

From the Kitchen of:

Recipe: _______________________

Serving: _______________   Prep Time: _______________

Cook Time: _______________   Temperature: _______________

Ingredients:

____

____

____

____

____

____

____

____

____

____

____

____

____

Methods:

____

____

____

____

____

____

____

____

____

____

____

____

____

Wine Pairing: _______________________

From the Kitchen of: _______________________

Recipe:

Serving: Prep Time:

Cook Time: Temperature:

Ingredients: Methods:

Wine Pairing:

From the Kitchen of:

Recipe:

Serving: Prep Time:

Cook Time: Temperature:

Ingredients: Methods:

Wine Pairing:

From the Kitchen of:

Recipe: ___________________________

Serving: _____________   Prep Time: _____________

Cook Time: _____________   Temperature: _____________

Ingredients:

____

____

____

____

____

____

____

____

____

____

____

____

____

____

Methods:

____

____

____

____

____

____

____

____

____

____

____

____

____

____

Wine Pairing: ___________________________

From the Kitchen of: ___________________________

Recipe:

Serving: Prep Time:

Cook Time: Temperature:

Ingredients: Methods:

Wine Pairing:

From the Kitchen of:

Smoothies

Recipe:

Serving:

Prep Time:

Cook Time:

Temperature:

Ingredients:

Methods:

Wine Pairing:

From the Kitchen of:

Recipe:

Serving: Prep Time:

Cook Time: Temperature:

Ingredients: Methods:

Wine Pairing:

From the Kitchen of:

Recipe:

Serving: Prep Time:

Cook Time: Temperature:

Ingredients: Methods:

Wine Pairing:

From the Kitchen of:

Recipe:

Serving: ___________   Prep Time: ___________

Cook Time: ___________   Temperature: ___________

Ingredients:

Methods:

Wine Pairing:

From the Kitchen of:

Recipe:

Serving: Prep Time:

Cook Time: Temperature:

Ingredients: Methods:

Wine Pairing:

From the Kitchen of:

Recipe:

Serving:

Prep Time:

Cook Time:

Temperature:

Ingredients:

Methods:

Wine Pairing:

From the Kitchen of:

Recipe:

Serving: Prep Time:

Cook Time: Temperature:

Ingredients: Methods:

Wine Pairing:

From the Kitchen of:

Recipe:

Serving: Prep Time:

Cook Time: Temperature:

Ingredients: Methods:

Wine Pairing:

From the Kitchen of:

Recipe:

Serving:

Prep Time:

Cook Time:

Temperature:

Ingredients:

Methods:

Wine Pairing:

From the Kitchen of:

Snacks

Recipe: ___________________________

Serving: _______________   Prep Time: _______________

Cook Time: _______________   Temperature: _______________

Ingredients:

____

____

____

____

____

____

____

____

____

____

____

____

____

____

Methods:

____

____

____

____

____

____

____

____

____

____

____

____

____

____

Wine Pairing: _______________________________________

From the Kitchen of: _______________________________________

Recipe: _______________________________

Serving: _______________   Prep Time: _______________

Cook Time: _______________   Temperature: _______________

Ingredients:

Methods:

Wine Pairing: _______________________________

From the Kitchen of: _______________________________

Recipe:

Serving:

Prep Time:

Cook Time:

Temperature:

Ingredients:

Methods:

Wine Pairing:

From the Kitchen of:

Recipe:

Serving: Prep Time:

Cook Time: Temperature:

Ingredients: Methods:

Wine Pairing:

From the Kitchen of:

Recipe:

Serving: Prep Time:

Cook Time: Temperature:

Ingredients: Methods:

Wine Pairing:

From the Kitchen of:

Recipe:

Serving:

Prep Time:

Cook Time:

Temperature:

Ingredients:

Methods:

Wine Pairing:

From the Kitchen of:

Recipe: ___________________________

Serving: ___________   Prep Time: ___________

Cook Time: ___________   Temperature: ___________

Ingredients:

_______________________   Methods:

____

_______________________   _______________________

_______________________   _______________________

_______________________   _______________________

_______________________   _______________________

_______________________   _______________________

_______________________   _______________________

_______________________   _______________________

_______________________   _______________________

_______________________   _______________________

_______________________   _______________________

_______________________   _______________________

_______________________   _______________________

_______________________   _______________________

Wine Pairing: ___________________________

From the Kitchen of: ___________________________

Recipe:

Serving:

Prep Time:

Cook Time:

Temperature:

Ingredients:

Methods:

Wine Pairing:

From the Kitchen of:

Recipe:

Serving:

Prep Time:

Cook Time:

Temperature:

Ingredients:

Methods:

Wine Pairing:

From the Kitchen of:

Soups

Recipe:

Serving:

Prep Time:

Cook Time:

Temperature:

Ingredients:

Methods:

Wine Pairing:

From the Kitchen of:

Recipe:

Serving: Prep Time:

Cook Time: Temperature:

Ingredients: Methods:

Wine Pairing:

From the Kitchen of:

Recipe:

Serving:

Prep Time:

Cook Time:

Temperature:

Ingredients:

Methods:

Wine Pairing:

From the Kitchen of:

Recipe:

Serving: Prep Time:

Cook Time: Temperature:

Ingredients: Methods:

Wine Pairing:

From the Kitchen of:

Recipe:

Serving:

Prep Time:

Cook Time:

Temperature:

Ingredients:

Methods:

Wine Pairing:

From the Kitchen of:

Recipe:

Serving:

Prep Time:

Cook Time:

Temperature:

Ingredients:

Methods:

Wine Pairing:

From the Kitchen of:

Recipe:

Serving:

Prep Time:

Cook Time:

Temperature:

Ingredients:

Methods:

Wine Pairing:

From the Kitchen of:

Recipe: ___________________________

Serving: ___________   Prep Time: ___________

Cook Time: ___________   Temperature: ___________

Ingredients:

____
____
____
____
____
____
____
____
____
____
____
____
____
____

Methods:

____
____
____
____
____
____
____
____
____
____
____
____
____
____

Wine Pairing: ___________________________

From the Kitchen of: ___________________________

Recipe: _______________________________

Serving: _______________   Prep Time: _______________

Cook Time: _______________   Temperature: _______________

Ingredients: Methods:

_______________________   _______________________

_______________________   _______________________

_______________________   _______________________

_______________________   _______________________

_______________________   _______________________

_______________________   _______________________

_______________________   _______________________

_______________________   _______________________

_______________________   _______________________

_______________________   _______________________

_______________________   _______________________

_______________________   _______________________

_______________________   _______________________

_______________________   _______________________

_______________________   _______________________

Wine Pairing: _______________________________

From the Kitchen of: _______________________________

Sauces

Recipe:

Serving: ___________   Prep Time: ___________

Cook Time: ___________   Temperature: ___________

Ingredients: Methods:

Wine Pairing:

From the Kitchen of:

Recipe: ______________________________

Serving: ______________ Prep Time: ______________

Cook Time: ______________ Temperature: ______________

Ingredients:

____
____
____
____
____
____
____
____
____
____
____
____
____
____
____

Methods:

____
____
____
____
____
____
____
____
____
____
____
____
____
____
____

Wine Pairing: ______________________________

From the Kitchen of: ______________________________

Recipe:

Serving: Prep Time:

Cook Time: Temperature:

Ingredients: Methods:

Wine Pairing:

From the Kitchen of:

Recipe:

Serving: Prep Time:

Cook Time: Temperature:

Ingredients: Methods:

Wine Pairing:

From the Kitchen of:

Recipe:

Serving:

Prep Time:

Cook Time:

Temperature:

Ingredients:

Methods:

Wine Pairing:

From the Kitchen of:

Recipe:

Serving: Prep Time:

Cook Time: Temperature:

Ingredients: Methods:

Wine Pairing:

From the Kitchen of:

Recipe:

Serving: Prep Time:

Cook Time: Temperature:

Ingredients: Methods:

Wine Pairing:

From the Kitchen of:

Recipe:

Serving: Prep Time:

Cook Time: Temperature:

Ingredients: Methods:

Wine Pairing:

From the Kitchen of:

Recipe:

Serving:

Prep Time:

Cook Time:

Temperature:

Ingredients:

Methods:

Wine Pairing:

From the Kitchen of:

Salads

Recipe:

Serving: Prep Time:

Cook Time: Temperature:

Ingredients: Methods:

Wine Pairing:

From the Kitchen of:

Recipe:

Serving: Prep Time:

Cook Time: Temperature:

Ingredients: Methods:

Wine Pairing:

From the Kitchen of:

Recipe:

Serving: Prep Time:

Cook Time: Temperature:

Ingredients: Methods:

Wine Pairing:

From the Kitchen of:

Recipe:

Serving:

Prep Time:

Cook Time:

Temperature:

Ingredients:

Methods:

Wine Pairing:

From the Kitchen of:

Recipe:

Serving: Prep Time:

Cook Time: Temperature:

Ingredients: Methods:

Wine Pairing:

From the Kitchen of:

Recipe:

Serving: Prep Time:

Cook Time: Temperature:

Ingredients: Methods:

Wine Pairing:

From the Kitchen of:

Recipe:

Serving: Prep Time:

Cook Time: Temperature:

Ingredients: Methods:

Wine Pairing:

From the Kitchen of:

Recipe:

Serving: Prep Time:

Cook Time: Temperature:

Ingredients: Methods:

Wine Pairing:

From the Kitchen of:

Recipe:

Serving: ___________ Prep Time: ___________

Cook Time: ___________ Temperature: ___________

Ingredients: **Methods:**

Wine Pairing: ___________

From the Kitchen of: ___________

Dips

Recipe:

Serving: Prep Time:

Cook Time: Temperature:

Ingredients: Methods:

Wine Pairing:

From the Kitchen of:

Recipe: ______________________________

Serving: ______________   Prep Time: ______________

Cook Time: ______________   Temperature: ______________

Ingredients: Methods:

____________________   ____________________

____________________   ____________________

____________________   ____________________

____________________   ____________________

____________________   ____________________

____________________   ____________________

____________________   ____________________

____________________   ____________________

____________________   ____________________

____________________   ____________________

____________________   ____________________

____________________   ____________________

____________________   ____________________

____________________   ____________________

Wine Pairing: ______________________________

From the Kitchen of: ______________________________

Recipe:

Serving: Prep Time:

Cook Time: Temperature:

Ingredients: Methods:

Wine Pairing:

From the Kitchen of:

Recipe:

Serving:

Prep Time:

Cook Time:

Temperature:

Ingredients:

Methods:

Wine Pairing:

From the Kitchen of:

Recipe:

Serving: ___________

Prep Time: ___________

Cook Time: ___________

Temperature: ___________

Ingredients:

____

____

____

____

____

____

____

____

____

____

____

____

____

____

Methods:

____

____

____

____

____

____

____

____

____

____

____

____

____

____

Wine Pairing: ___________

From the Kitchen of: ___________

Other Goodies

Recipe:

Serving: Prep Time:

Cook Time: Temperature:

Ingredients: Methods:

Wine Pairing:

From the Kitchen of:

Recipe:

Serving: Prep Time:

Cook Time: Temperature:

Ingredients: Methods:

Wine Pairing:

From the Kitchen of:

Recipe:

Serving: Prep Time:

Cook Time: Temperature:

Ingredients: Methods:

Wine Pairing:

From the Kitchen of:

Recipe:

Serving: Prep Time:

Cook Time: Temperature:

Ingredients: Methods:

Wine Pairing:

From the Kitchen of: